# The Adventures of
# Sydney and Jack

## Abigail Galas

PAGE PUBLISHING, INC.
Conneaut Lake, PA

First originally published by Page Publishing 2021

ISBN 978-1-6624-3942-1 (pbk)
ISBN 978-1-6624-3943-8 (digital)

Printed in the United States of America

# Dedication

I dedicate this book to the Leandro Family. You are a bright light and an inspiration. I am blessed to call you family.

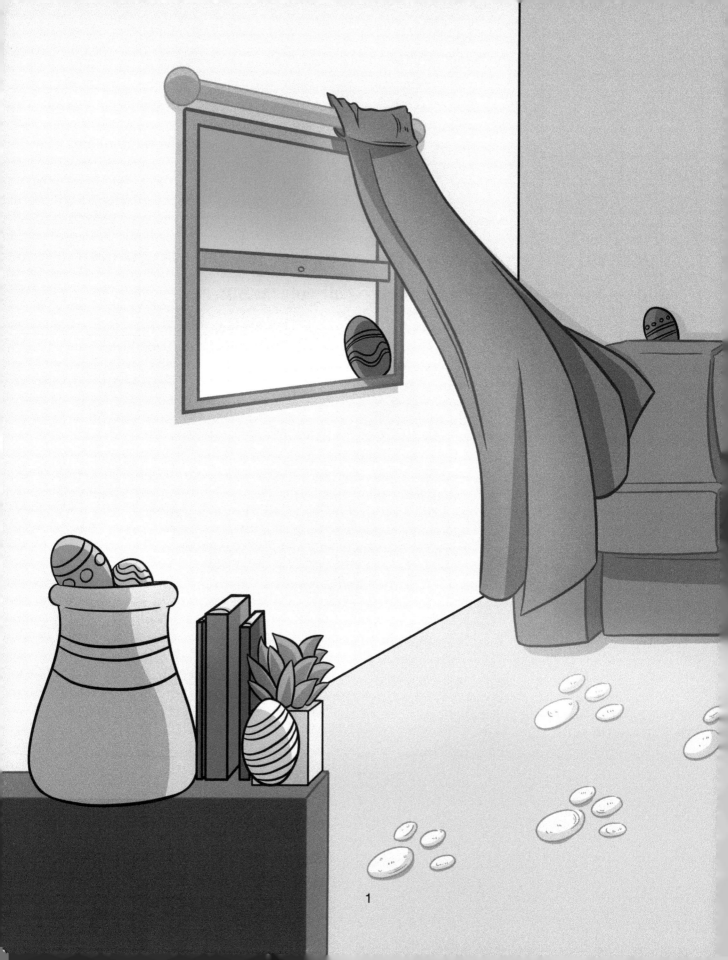

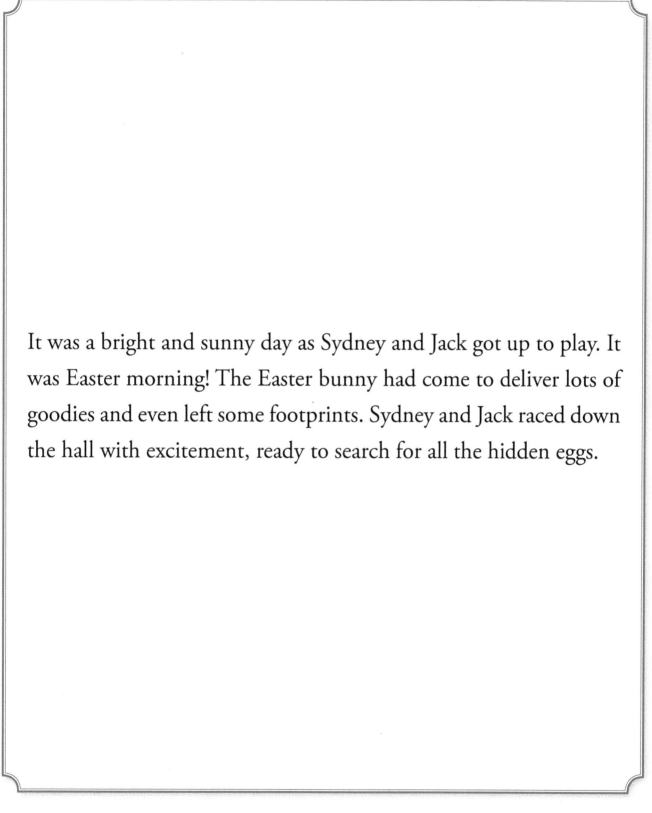

It was a bright and sunny day as Sydney and Jack got up to play. It was Easter morning! The Easter bunny had come to deliver lots of goodies and even left some footprints. Sydney and Jack raced down the hall with excitement, ready to search for all the hidden eggs.

"I found a pink egg!" yelled Sydney.

"And I found a red egg!" chorused Jack.

They went room to room searching high and low to collect every egg.

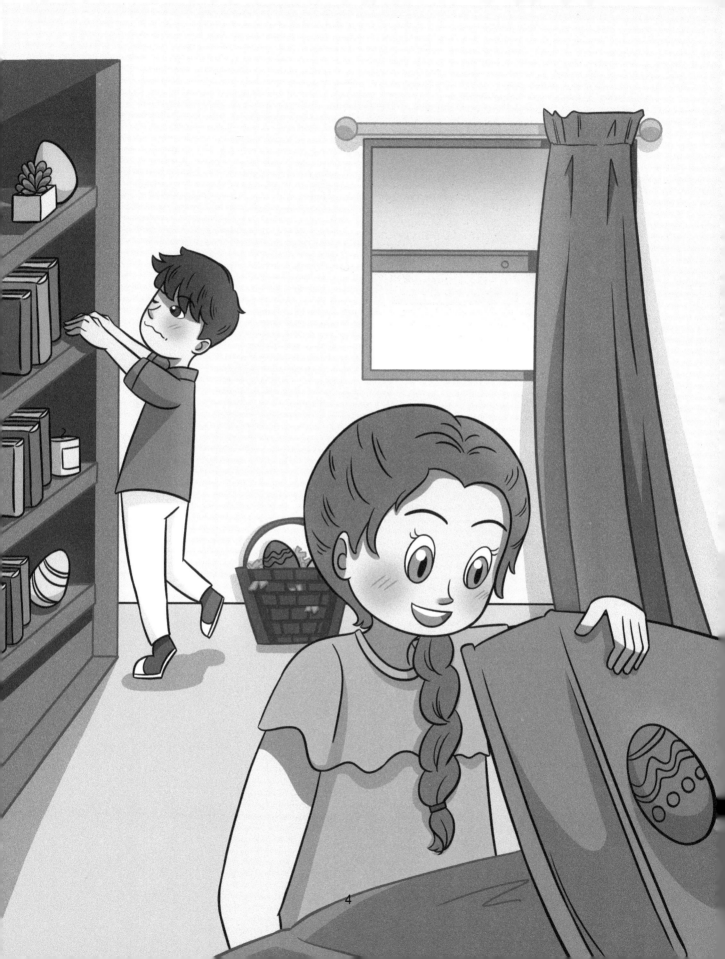

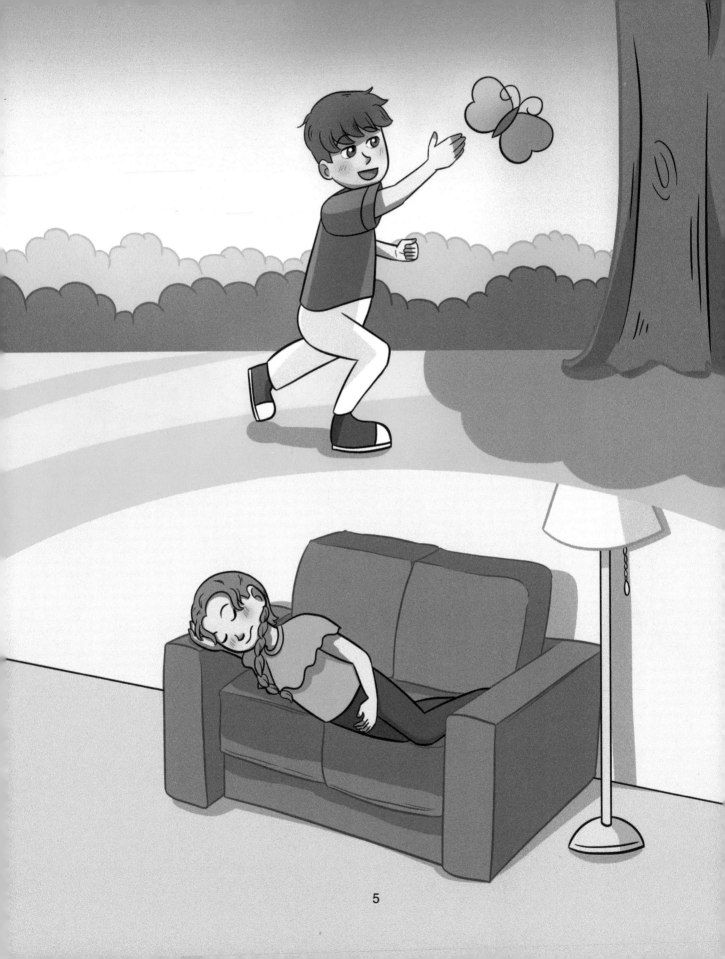

Once all the eggs were collected, Sydney became very tired and decided to lay on the couch while Jack was running and jumping outside.

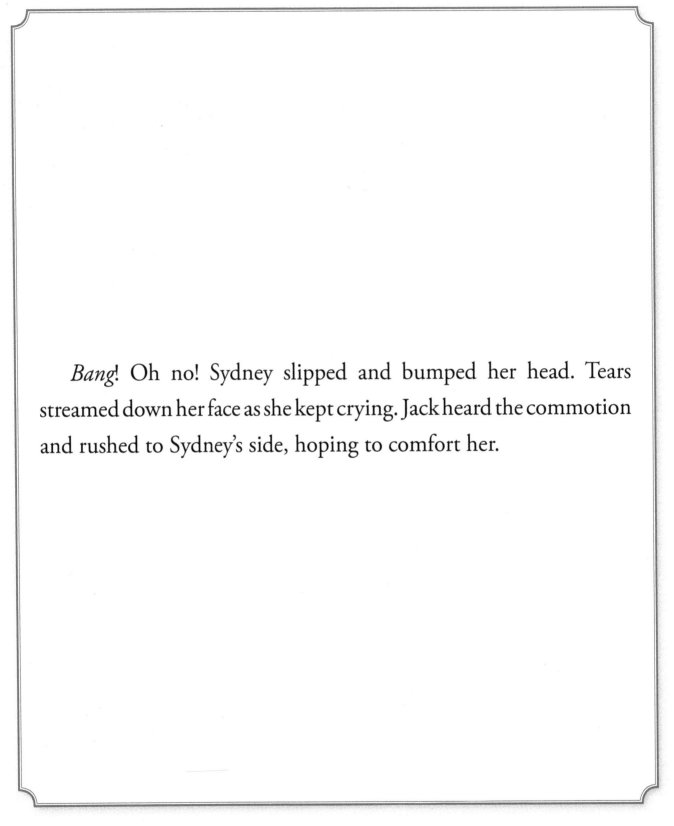

*Bang*! Oh no! Sydney slipped and bumped her head. Tears streamed down her face as she kept crying. Jack heard the commotion and rushed to Sydney's side, hoping to comfort her.

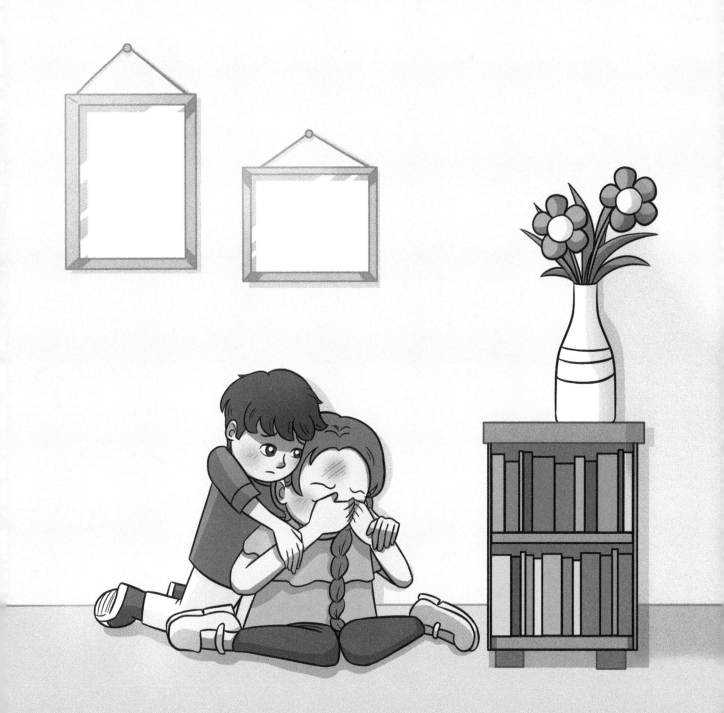

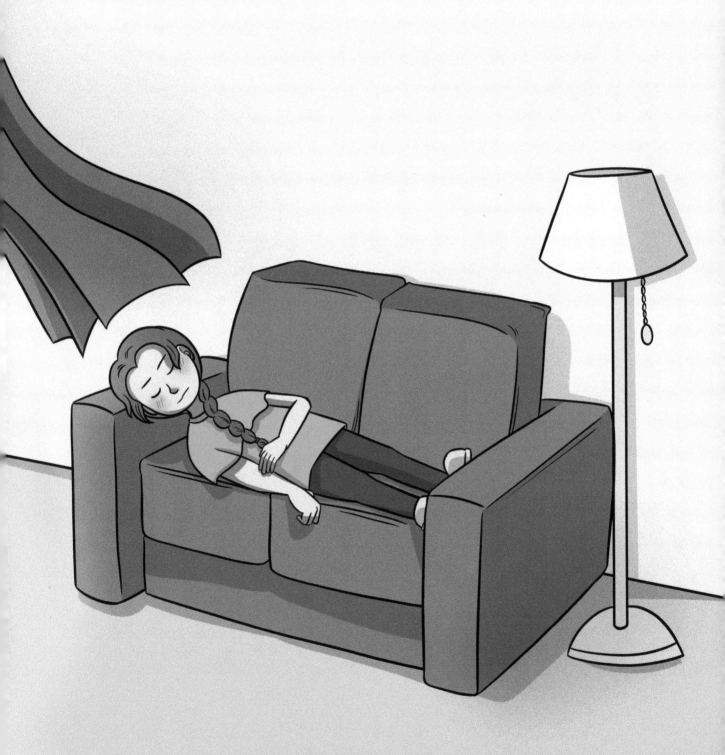

As the day wore on, Sydney became more and more tired. While family arrived, Sydney slept. While Easter lunch was being eaten, Sydney slept. While everyone went to enjoy the day outside, Sydney slept. Sydney could not seem to muster the energy for a play-filled Easter day. By 3:30 p.m., Sydney was exhausted, and it was decided she needed to visit the doctors. When Sydney arrived at the doctor, they told her she needed to go to the hospital for some tests. As Sydney arrived at the hospital, they brought her to her own room to start the first test.

They had to take some of Sydney's blood to test it and see what was making her feel sick and tired. When the test came back, the doctor had to send Sydney to another hospital in Boston for some more tests on her blood.

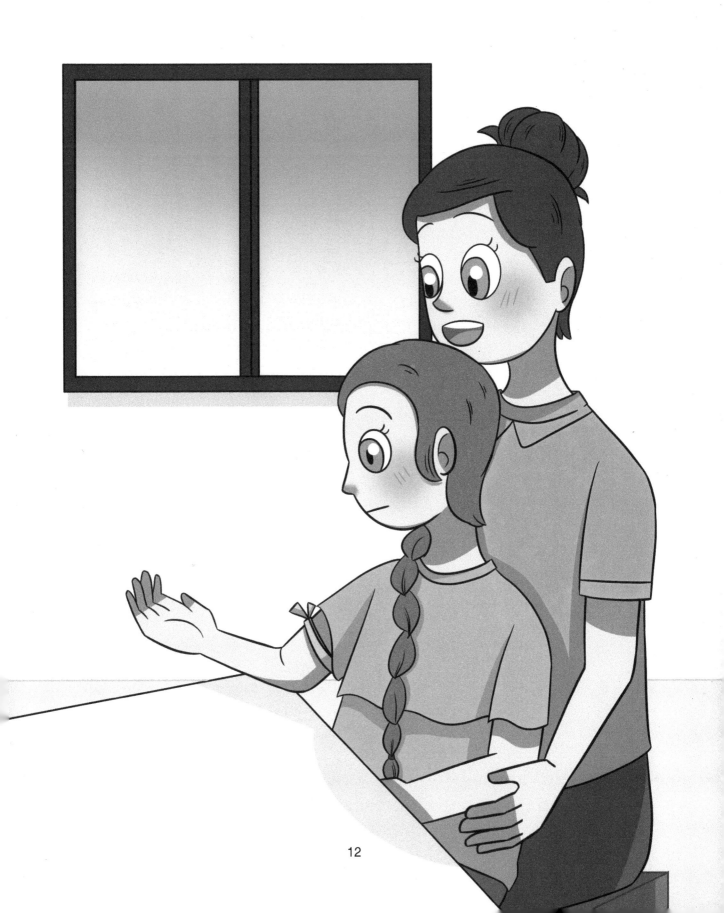

12

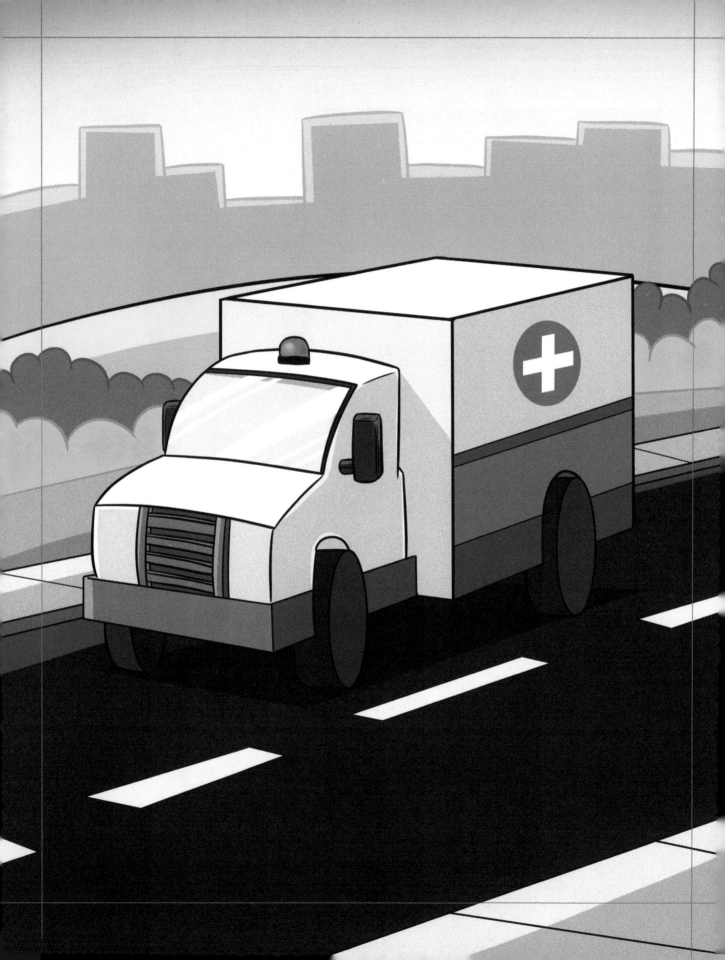

Sydney was taken to the new hospital by an ambulance with flashing lights and a loud siren. When Sydney arrived at the new hospital, her doctor and nurses ran some more tests on her blood. They told her she would have to stay the night while they waited for the results. Sydney and her family waited and waited and even waited some more to get the results.

When the results finally came, the doctor told Sydney's parents that she has a very bad disease called cancer. Sydney has what is known as B-cell acute lymphoblastic leukemia. This means she has cancer in her blood. For thirty-eight days, Sydney spent her days and nights in the hospital getting treatments known as chemo to help defeat her cancer.

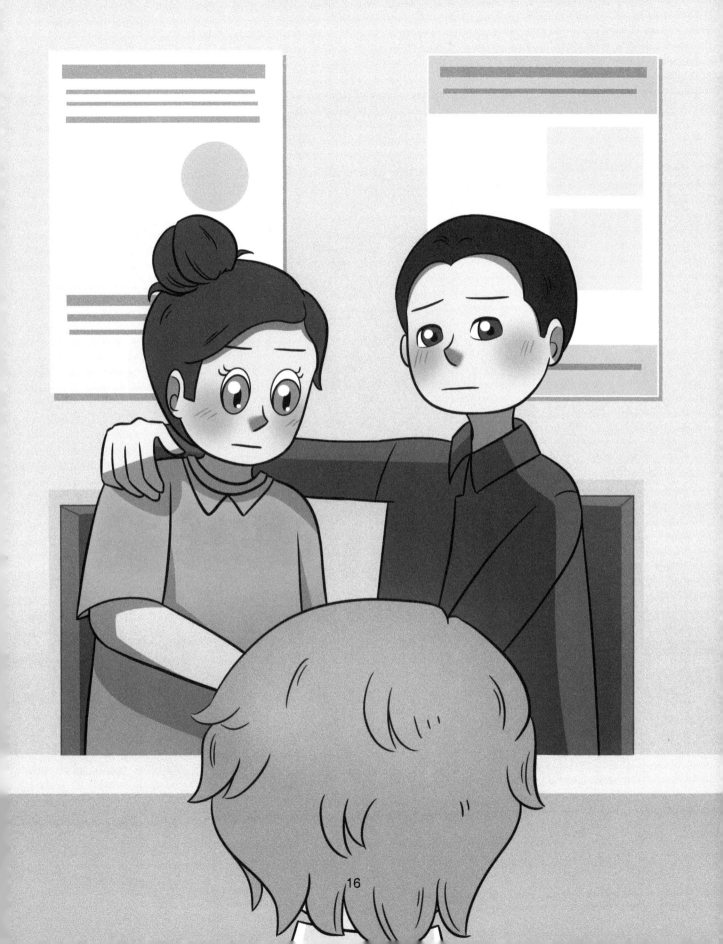

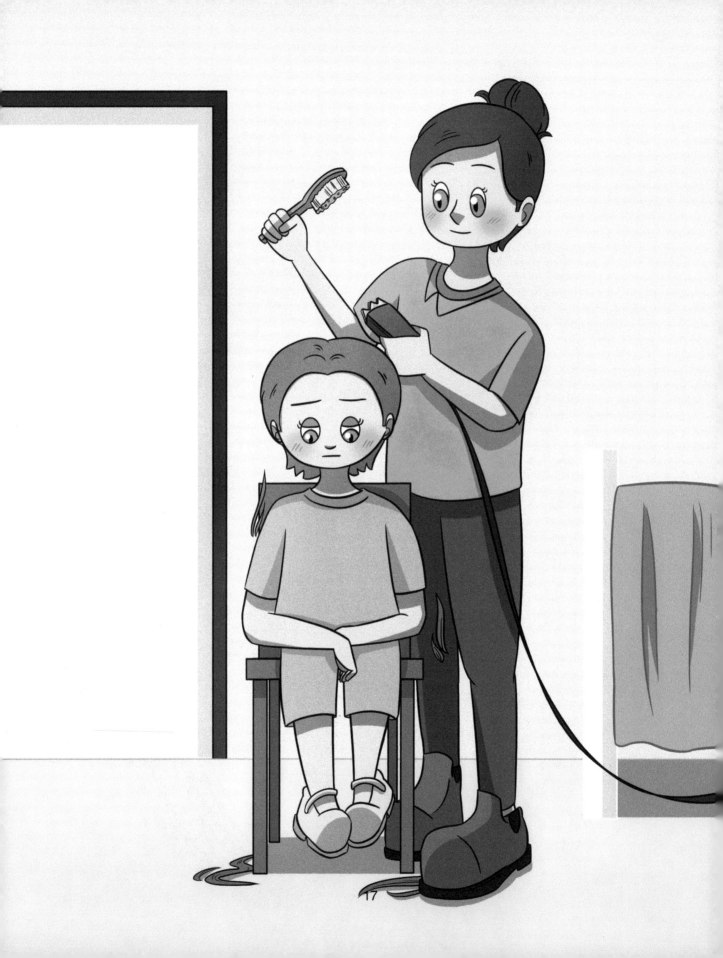

As she continued to get the medicine she needs, her hair started falling out, so she decided to shave it off.

"I'm like Daddy now!" Sydney exclaimed.

As the days in the hospital continued, Sydney received more chemo treatments and had many procedures done all to help her defeat this awful disease.

Finally, it was time Sydney could go back home. She will continue to receive chemo to battle her cancer, but she is a true fighter and a true hero. Sydney and Jack, your favorite duo, were back together and ready to take on anything.

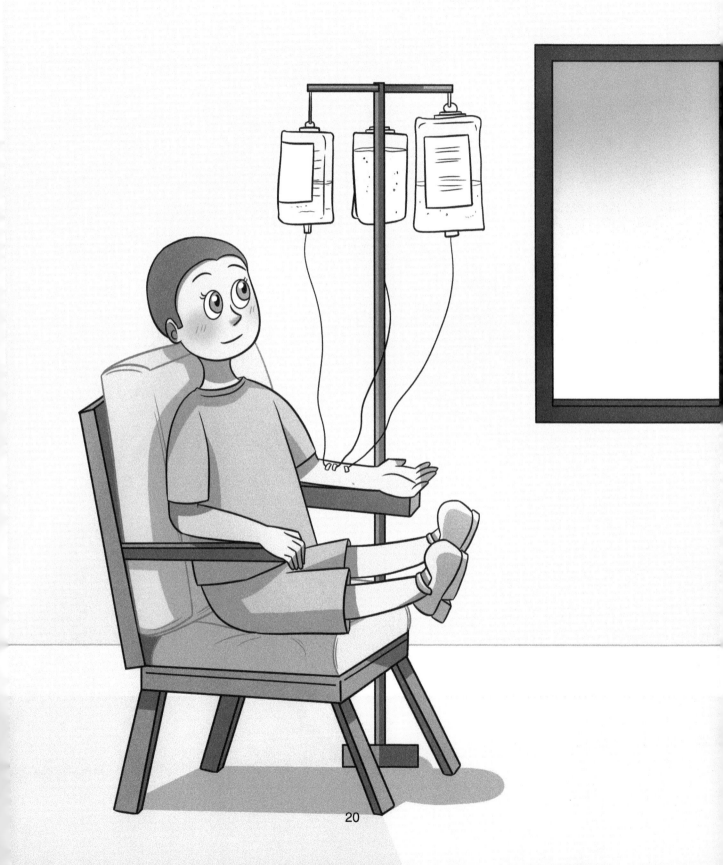

# Meet the Duo

SYDNEY. I am five years old, and I love gardening, playing with bubbles, and ballet. One day, I want to be a veterinarian. I am a brave, smart, beautiful little girl. I am compassionate, kind, and loving. I am a fighter!

JACK. I am three years old, and I love gardening, fishing, and dirt bikes. I am an energetic, strong, and courageous little boy. I am helpful, funny, and loving. I am my sister's best friend. I will help her fight!

# Message from Me

When I first heard of Sydney's diagnosis, I think I was in complete shock. I had known this amazing little girl from the preschool I work at and just couldn't believe the news. My family knows the word cancer all too well, but when I heard that Sydney was diagnosed with leukemia, I think it struck differently, knowing that this young child has a long fight ahead of her. In retrospect, I have always known about childhood cancer, but seeing it firsthand was completely different. It led to my doing more research and finding out that less than 4 percent of cancer research funds go to childhood cancer, so in writing this book, I pray to bring awareness to childhood cancer and let children that are facing cancer know they are not alone.

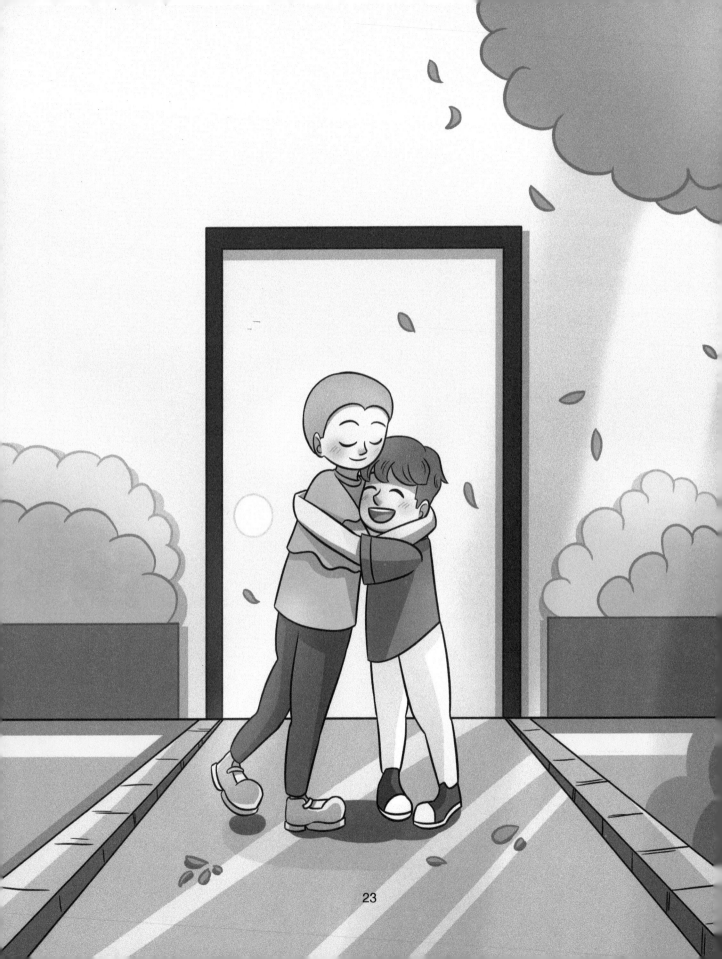

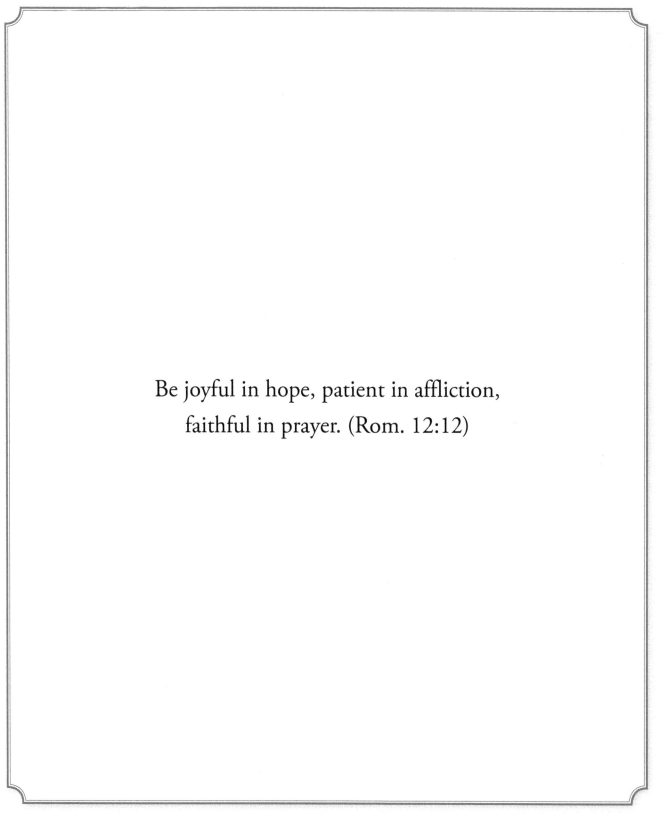

Be joyful in hope, patient in affliction,
faithful in prayer. (Rom. 12:12)

# About the Author

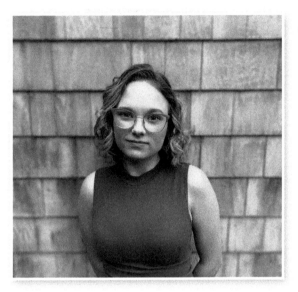

Abigail Galas is an aspiring author, hoping to help change the world one book at a time. She decided to write *The Adventures of Sydney and Jack* to bring awareness to Sydney's cancer journey and bring forth hope for all children fighting cancer. Galas knows firsthand the effects of cancer within her own family and wishes to bring awareness to the awful disease to promote an understanding and giving attitude to one day find a cure for all cancers. Galas enjoys some of her free time by reading, drawing, and having family movie nights. If you would like to know more about Galas, her upcoming books and events, you can find her at Instagram, @Author_ASG, and Facebook page, Abby Galas.